FIT through the CORONAVIRUS PANDEMIC
„INSIDER TIP" from a MEDIUM !
Tayala Léha

AF200564

FIT

through the

CORONAVIRUS PANDEMIC

"INSIDER TIP" from a MEDIUM!

Tayala Léha

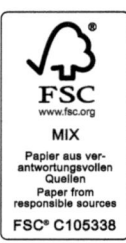

Note:

This book is printed in a larger font for greater readability.

Bibliographical information of the German National Library: The German National Library lists this publication in the German National Bibliography; detailed bibliographical information can be found on the internet at www.dnb.de.

© Text 2020 by Tayala Léha
All rights reserved.

Production and publication:
BoD - Books on Demand, Norderstedt

ISBN 978-3-7519-0495-7

Table of contents

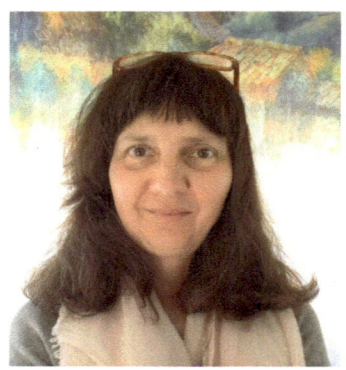

Preface

I'm Tayala Léha, a healer and author with the gift of medium since birth.

I'm writing this booklet in light of the current situation. I've been deeply affected by events surrounding the pandemic. I've asked IN PRAYER:

"What can we humans DO to protect ourselves?"

This booklet sheds light on the result.

It's not possible to avoid becoming infected. There's always a risk. But what matters is how the body COPES with the virus.

You might contract the virus and fall ill. What's important is preventing a fatal outcome as far as possible.

I myself safely received the message "from above". That's when I started writing the booklet. I also fell ill recently. I finished writing the booklet with a fever because it's important for me that the world sees it and it can help people.

Every "message from the UPPER WORLD" in my life has so far been correct.
I trust in them and, of course, practise what I preach. I've thoroughly researched whether the "INSIDER TIP" can be justified from a medical point of view. Not only was it justified, it was spot on!

I've written this booklet with the intention of sending HOPE into the world, because that's what we all need the most...
I wish you all strength in these challenging times.

With warmest wishes, Tayala Léha.

Is there a remedy for COVID-19?

It's usually just the stuff of films: an epidemic threatens humanity and there's no antidote. Then a "cure" is discovered and everyone gets better...

"Usually", we're delighted and turn the TV off. We're back in our safe world out of harm's way.

But today, the world's been turned upside down. We can't switch off, we can't ignore the death rates. The threat may still be a long way from us. But it can strike at any time - like it has me.

There's always HOPE. You just have to find a way. I've done it my own way and want to share my knowledge with you. Perhaps a glimmer of hope in these sad times, where despite everyone's best efforts, victory is still out of reach.

COVID-19 is now a harsh reality! But we should still remember: "For every disease, there is a herb to treat it...". Please read under "INSIDER TIP". All other measures help the cause...

Is there a remedy for COVID-19?

I really hope that I've shared it with you here!

Violet light

Colours have a special effect on the body and soul.

They emit specific frequencies that have different effects on us.

"RED LIGHT DISTRICT". Heard of it? There's a reason that RED is used in this line of work. It has a stimulating effect on both body and mind.

RED LIGHT at the traffic lights has a signal effect.

We now need something that acts as a disinfectant.

The effects of ultraviolet light for the purpose of disinfection are well established. But please don't use THAT. It can cause serious damage!

Instead, use **violet light**. It has an **ANTIVIRAL** effect and also acts as a disinfectant.

Flood your home with violet light!

Royal jelly

Royal jelly is secreted by honey bees to feed queen bees. It's an excellent tonic for humans too; after all, queen bees are only given the best.

Making a three-week cure with this valuable product is beneficial for us as it enhances the body's immune response...

What's more:
Experts considered royal jelly to be a highly effective, NATURAL antibiotic until penicillin was discovered. But it also actively combats VIRUSES, and its components are extremely valuable!

Please note!

If you're ALLERGIC to bee products, you should seek alternatives...

GOOD bacteria for the GUT

"Good" probiotic bacteria for the gut are vital for the correct functioning of our immune system. They can be taken as tablets or else there are powder products.

Lactobacillus acidophilus

Lactobacillus salivarius

Bifidobacterium longum

These are the THREE that you need in order to achieve the desired effect, namely STRENGTHENING!

This remedy is even more important if you've completed a course of antibiotics. If this is the case for you, it's vital you take it.

As simple as it sounds, it's very effective. But you also need a bit of patience: you should take it for at least 4 weeks to achieve the desired effect. Despite everything, it's worth taking it now.

The POWER of thought!

The power of thought! Imagine you're with your partner... come on, you know what I'm getting at... Not appropriate here? Oh, but it is, it's very appropriate here! To show you that sexual THOUGHTS leave behind "physical traces"... Our body reacts instantly to our thoughts. So be careful WHAT and HOW you think.

What's more: Athletes with injuries imagine completing their exercises – they think in precise IMAGES. It works and has been proven: training is only successful in thoughts!

PROTECTION starts in the mind. Think of boldly striding through the world, doing sport to keep fit and healthy, doing what makes you happy. And your body will gain only STRENGTH from these good thoughts but not trigger debilitating stress. But if you're permanently worrying and picturing the most awful scenarios, then... well, then unfortunately I can't help you with this booklet either. The only thing that helps is CHANGING HOW YOU THINK!

HEAT
to fight anxiety and panic

In Ayurveda, the mantra is: worries escalate if you don't ground yourself. Too many thoughts about one thing, too many worries - they quickly mount to become a "mental hurricane" that's out of control. What can we do?

Below are a few ideas for home that anyone can try. Such simple ideas to combat anxiety? Yes!

- warm salt foot baths in the evening
- warm baths
- eat lots of warm food and drink lots of warm drinks
- go to bed at a regular time
- everything in moderation: both your use of media and sleep
- choose stews over crispbread: opt for "liquid food" and avoid dry snacks...
- treat yourself to oil massages: from head to toe - highly effective, whether you're with your partner or own your own.

Japanese healing art:
Jin Shin Jyutsu

We all have vital energy, otherwise we wouldn't be here at all. It's very useful to activate or harmonise this vital energy if it's blocked, either by physical weaknesses or negative emotions!

Below are two important actions:

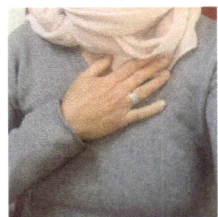

1. Place your hand onto the middle of your chest and leave it there until it "pulses".
2. Use your other hand to cover each individual finger and hold the finger until it starts to pulse. The vital energy then flows freely again. And this strengthens your immune system when you're suffering from negative thoughts, worries, anxiety, anger and also in general! Want to help someone far away? Place your hand onto a photo and "flow"!

Early to bed!

My grandmother used to say: "Go to bed early, sleep BEFORE midnight is best!"

When I was young, I used to think: "What nonsense!" But now I know she was right!

This applies to people who like to go to bed early and get up early.

What applies to all of us is that we all need sleep in times of stress and change, and enough of it. Too much screen time makes it difficult to sleep. Don't drive yourself crazy with the news. Listen to it, but turn it off early enough in the evening.

Sleep is vital for our health! Make sure you get enough of it to keep your strength up!

BREATHING!

Breathing's not just good, it's essential... Joking aside. Taking in a deep breath is relaxing.

Special forces are specially trained in breathing in stressful situations, because when you're scared, you breath quickly and don't take in much air. But this impairs important decision making that may be vital for saving your own life or that of your comrades.

Breathing PROPERLY means you can let go of worries. How?

Take a DEEP BREATH IN! And then slowly exhale, listening to the air being released. If you now do that 3 times, can you notice a difference from before?

It's been proven that paying attention to your breathing in stressful situations works. So be more aware of taking in a deep breath. It's worth it, both for your brain and your body!

GARLIC

Garlic smells. Let's be honest, it stinks. But: it's super healthy!

It's said to have both an ANTIVIRAL as well as an antibacterial EFFECT.

Eat it raw or add it to your cooking. Don't cook it for too long ideally. This can destroy the active ingredients.

I add it to anchovies – on its own. It's a healthy mixture.

Don't worry about your partner's sense of smell... ;)
Encourage them to eat garlic too, then you'll both stink against the rest of the world...

In the wake of the COVID-19 outbreak, China has distributed large amounts of garlic for free, according to the news. This has been ridiculed online in the "Western medical sector". Well, as far as I'M concerned, the Chinese are smart!

ONIONS

"The onion is worth as much as a whole pharmacy...", Paracelsus, a Swiss doctor and natural philosopher, once said about this very unremarkable vegetable.

The truth is that it also has an **antiviral** and antibacterial effect, just like garlic.

If you don't want to eat it (it works best when raw), then slice it up and put it next to your bed. The "vapours" keep the lungs free, making it easier to breath.

Legend has it that during the flu epidemic in 1919, there was a farming family that didn't fall ill. The woman had covered the whole house in onions and the doctor was able to prove by means of a microscopic examination that the virus had become attached to the onions' layers.

In the current climate, I now put a chopped-up onion next to my bed every evening.

UNSATURATED FATTY ACIDS

Fish oil capsules are useful for those who don't consume enough unsaturated fatty acids.

Fish oil has a very special composition: **EPA and DHA.** It is vital not to deprive the body of either fatty acid. A hundred years ago, we consumed substantially more unsaturated fatty acids than saturated. This made us healthier!

Important:
In the case of inflammatory diseases, the inflammation tendency can be reduced with a high dose of omega-3 fatty acids - perhaps not overnight, but it still works. **Fish oil therefore has anti-inflammatory properties!** And that may be beneficial to us now faced with this situation!

Unsaturated fatty acids also protect our blood vessels and heart.

In the case of multiple sclerosis, a modern-day scourge, it should be possible to successfully stem the inflammatory processes on the myelin sheaths (myelin sheaths are the tissue insulating the nerves). Owing to the current prevalence of this disease, I thought this was worth mentioning.

In the case of emotional stress and depression, the abovementioned, highly useful omega-3 fatty acids can have a **positive** effect on **mood**, which is perhaps not to be scoffed at after all in the context of continuing restrictions on going out...

Linseed oil is an alternative for vegans...
My grandfather always used to pour linseed oil onto his plate, sprinkle a little salt over it and then dip a bread roll in, which he heartily ate. He always claimed it was healthy. He ate it every day.
I didn't find the taste very appealing and didn't understand what the fuss was about.

Today I know that **linseed oil and fish oil** are a great way to keep your immune system intact thanks to their **long-chain omega-3 fatty acids**!

"INSIDER TIP!"

My "insider tip" on the topic of COVID-19
is:

TURMERIC!

Turmeric is usually just known as a spice
you can get at the supermarket. And yet it
can dye so much more than just food
yellow.

By the way, the monks in Tibet also take
advantage of this property to give their
robes their beautiful orange-yellow colour
just by using turmeric.

TURMERIC is one of the most powerful
antioxidants there is. It contains the active
substance, curcumin, and other different
substances, and what should really
interest us today is

IT HAS AN ANTIVIRAL EFFECT!

In Ayurveda, it is known as the "golden
root" and is a traditional remedy in
Ayurvedic medicine.
It is also occasionally used as a natural
antibiotic.

Now the important bit:

Its **ANTI-INFLAMMATORY PROPERTIES** prove their worth when used for pulmonary diseases that are the result of inflammatory processes. This includes virtually all respiratory diseases caused by bacteria and viruses.

In the case of COVID-19, fatal breathing problems are triggered by lung inflammation that is usually on both sides!

You should consume turmeric in high doses (2 to 4 tea spoons or even more) together with oily foods as turmeric is fat-soluble.
A dash of cayenne pepper should greatly increase the intake of the active substance, curcumin. Then add a bit of Vitamin C and honey to re-energise the defence cells!

By the way, the bulb is also considered to have an anti-aging effect.

For those taking blood-thinning medication:

PLEASE ALWAYS consult your doctor BEFORE CONSUMING large amounts of TURMERIC!

Care should also be taken if you have gallstones and/or inflammation of the bile duct and the gastrointestinal tract!

+++

Finally, I'd like to take this opportunity to share with you what struck me the most during my research of the specialist literature:

namely, **the use of turmeric in the field of inflammatory respiratory diseases should considerably reduce the mortality** (i.e. the death rate)!

If that's not a sign of hope, I don't know what is...!

+++

AFTERWORD

Dear reader, I would be so happy if help were to come from the plant world, because as my grandmother used to say: "For every disease, there is a herb to treat it...".

May this information bring hope to the world and to people and, personally, I'm not only regularly consuming large amounts of turmeric, but I am, of course, also practising all the other tips in quarantine that I recommend to you... ALL of them were sent to me in prayer, but first and foremost: TURMERIC!

I hope that you all maintain your strength and remain in good health, or else have a speedy recovery - and I extend that wish to everyone in the whole world!

Yours, Tayala Léha.

Recommended reading

This booklet is also available
in a German print edition.

ISBN 978-3-7504-8150-3

It is available in book stores in
Germany, Austria and Switzerland
as well as in England, Australia,
Canada and the USA.